SIMPLIFIED VENTILATORS

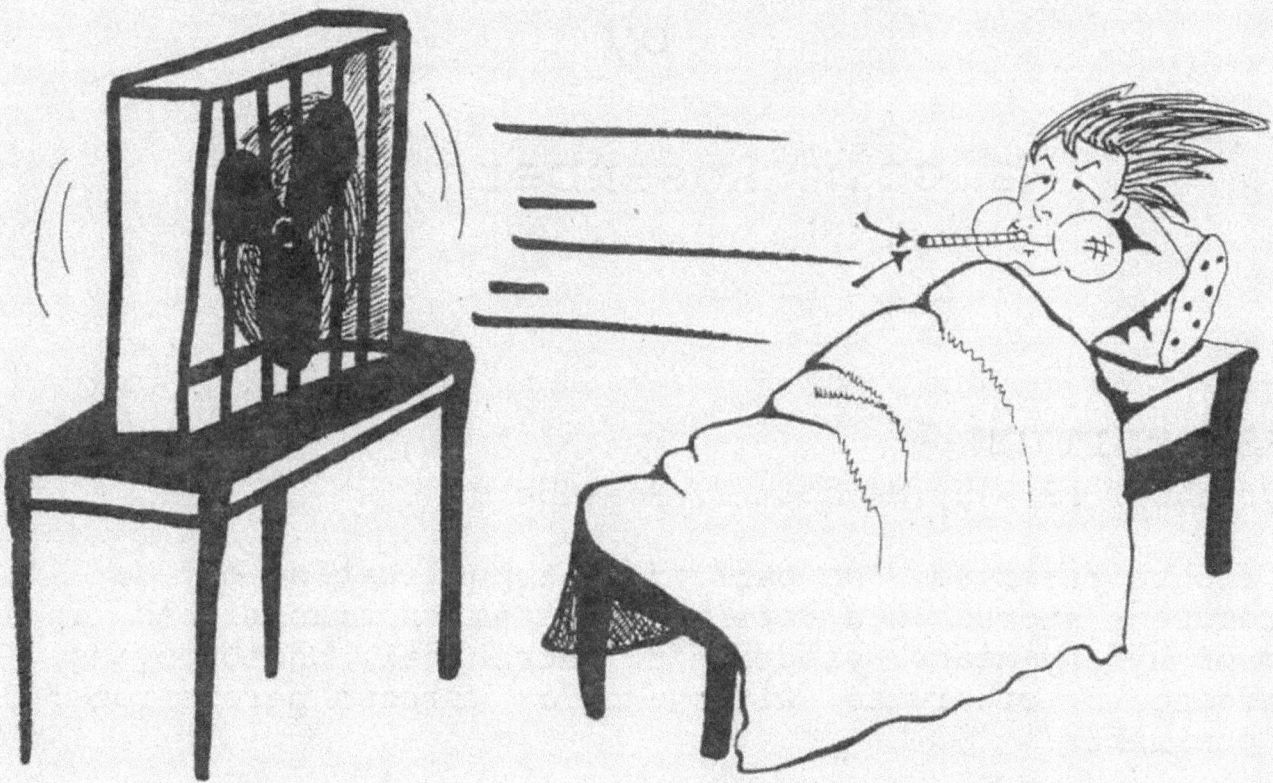

Malcolm Rosenberg, R. N.

Illustrations by Scott Brown

SIMPLIFIED VENTILATORS

by

Malcolm Rosenberg, R.N.

FIRST EDITION
Copyright © 1996 by Malcolm S. Rosenberg

Malcom Rosenberg
370 N.W. 115 Way
Coral Springs, FL 3071
(954) 753-5915

Copyrighted 1996
Printed in the United States of America

VENTILATORS

Ventilators are quite simple.
They are air pumps. Very similar to
the air pump for your bike.

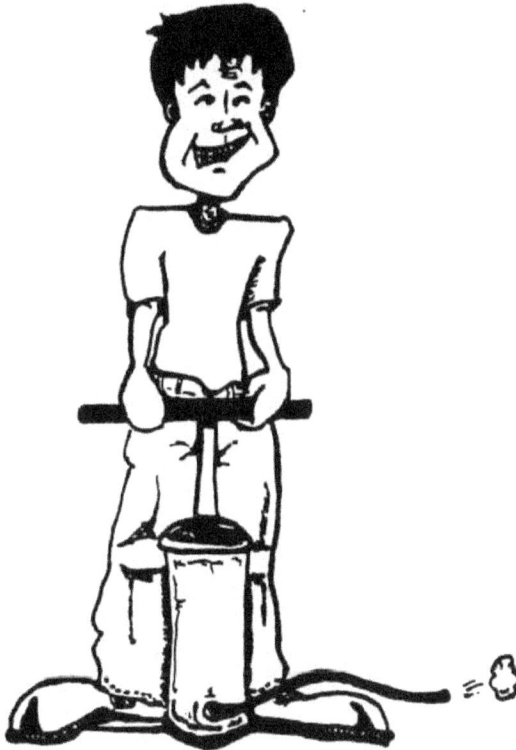

If you had the time and hand strength,
you could be a mechanical ventilator.

Tidal Volume

In the case of a ventilator, tidal volume is the amount of air pumped each stroke. If we breathe normally, tidal volume is what we normally inhale.

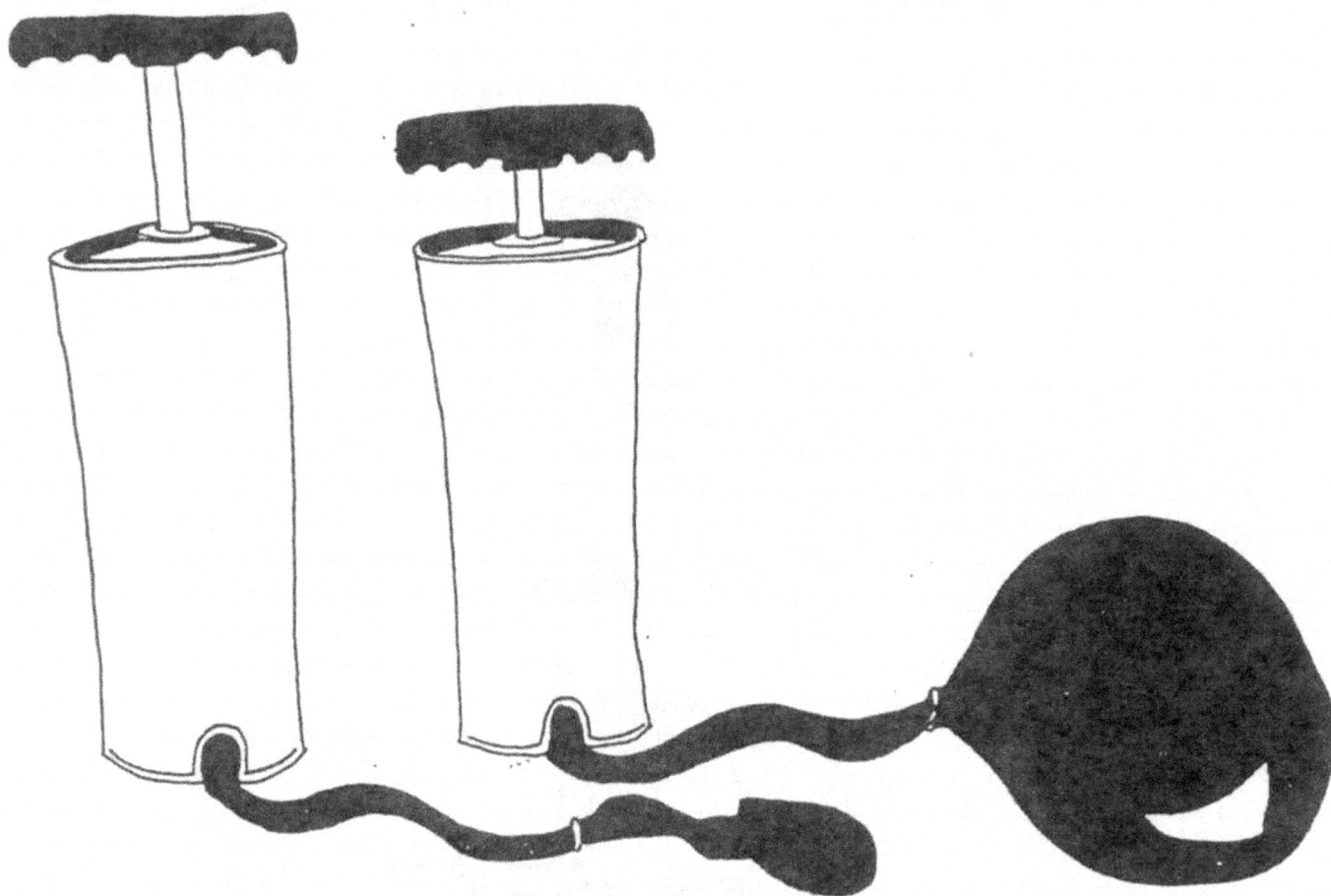

The balloon is like your lungs. How much it inflates is the tidal volume.

FiO₂

FiO$_2$ is the percentage of air that is oxygen that the

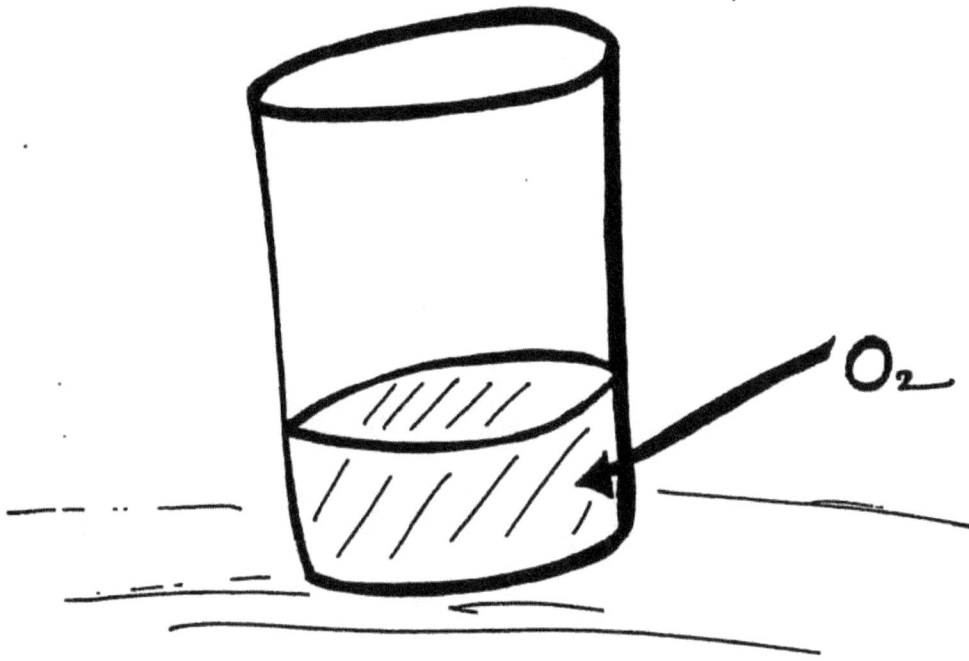

ventilator delivers. Atmospheric air (which most of us breathe) is 21% O$_2$. A ventilator can change the percentage. The normal range is 30% to 40%.

ASSIST CONTROL (AC)

Assist control means the machine gives the patient the number of breaths ordered (AC 16, AC 12, or whatever number at the tidal volume ordered).

Let's say 12

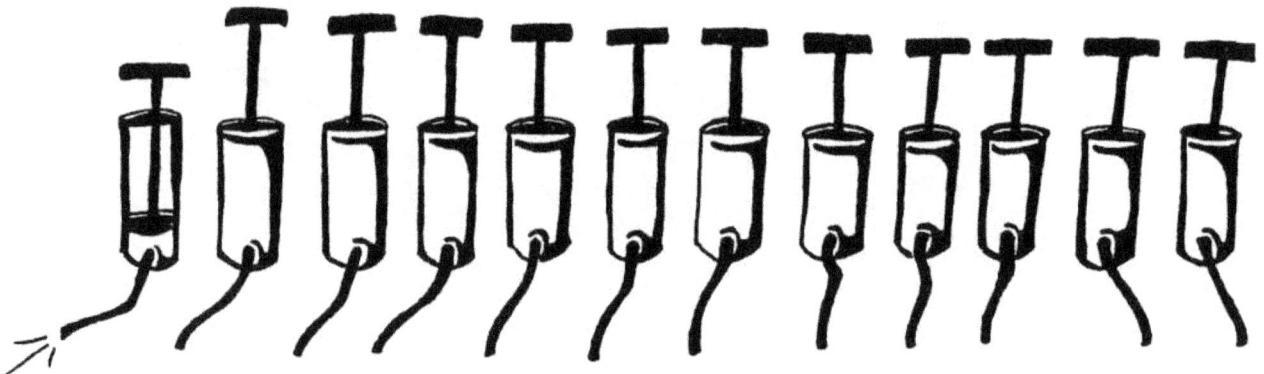

The ventilator will deliver 12 breaths at 5 second intervals (60/12 = 5).

In between those machine
breaths the patient can
initiate breaths. If the
patient inhales just the
tiniest little

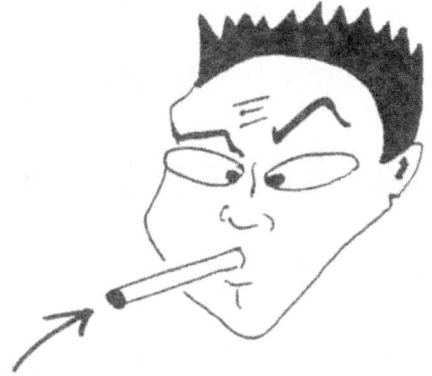

bit the machine will
deliver a full breath
at the set tidal volume.

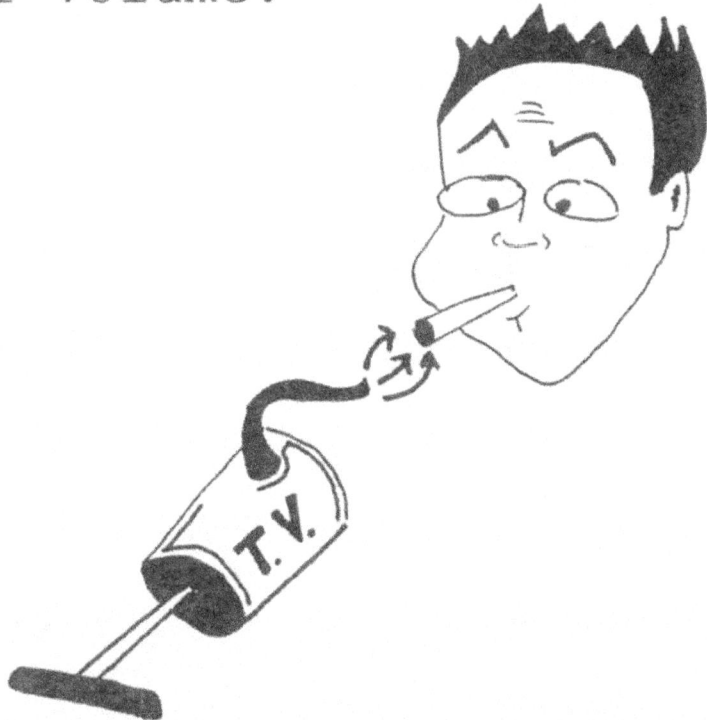

The other feature of assist control is that the ventilator will deliver a full tidal volume if inhaled the slightest bit.

If the patient **initiates** 5 breaths, he will **get** 5 breaths between those set 12 assisted breaths.

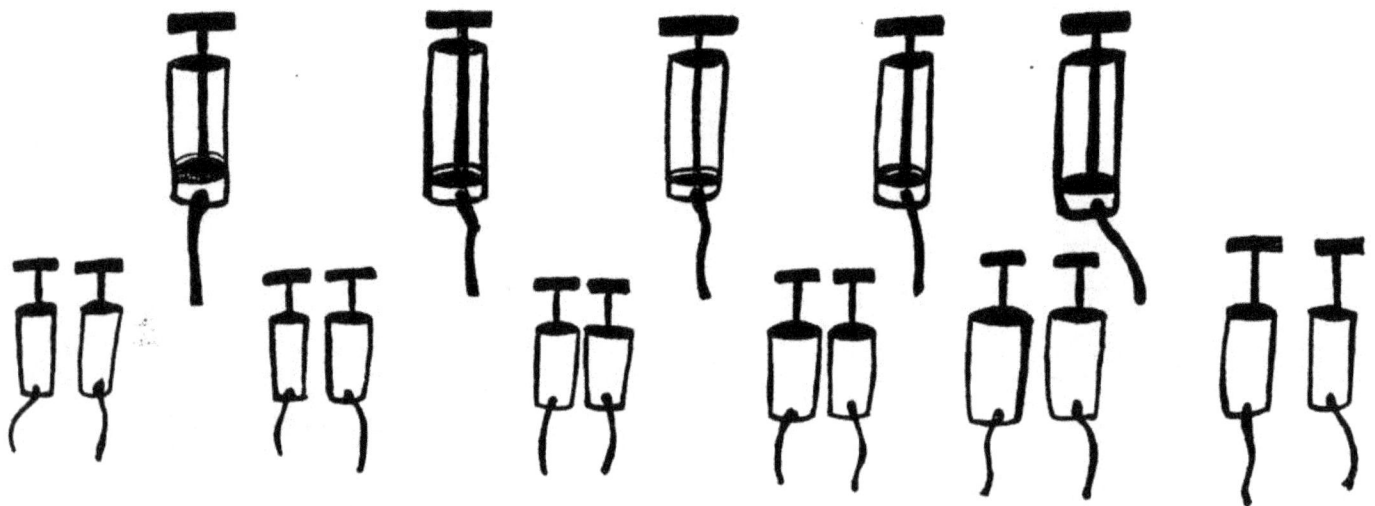

In assist control the machine does all the work. If the patient wants more air the machine will give it - <u>with no more work.</u>

SIMV

Synchronized Intermittent Mandatory Ventilation

Like assist control, "SIMV" or "IMV" is always ordered with a number (i.e. "SIMV 12" or "SIMV 2").

Like assist control, that number is how many forced breaths (mandatory breaths) the machine will deliver. "SIMV 12" means the machine will deliver 12 breaths at the set tidal volume.

The "SI" in SIMV is not *Sports Illustrated*. It is the abbreviation for "synchronized intermittent." That means the person can breathe on their own in between the machine breaths. The patient can breathe as **often** as they want and as **much** as they want. The patient can breathe at their own **rate** and **tidal volume**.

Let's look at SIMV 12 (or more commonly said, "IMV 12") at a tidal volume of 750. The machine will deliver the 12 mandatory ventilation's ("MV").

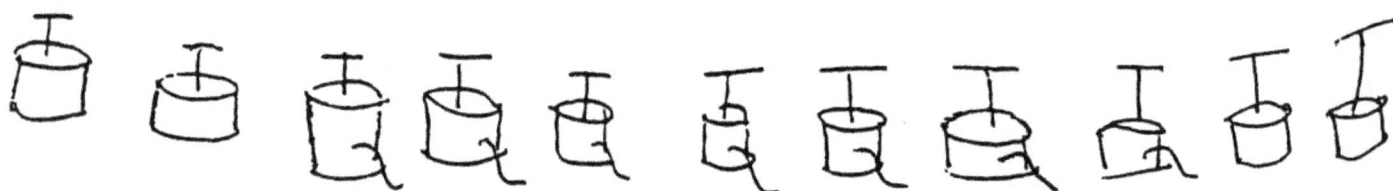

If the patient wants more air he has to breathe on his own and can inhale as much or as little as he wants. That is **the** difference between assist control and IMV. On IMV the patient must expend the energy to breathe extra.

Here we see 6 extra breaths of 500cc, 800cc, 300cc, 400cc, 600cc, and 500cc

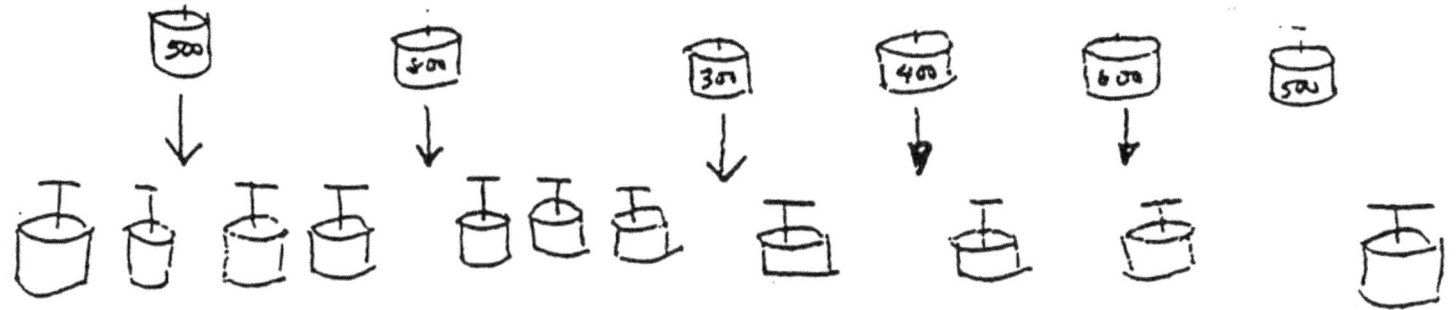

in between the 12 mandated breaths of 700cc. They are not machine delivered. So I didn't draw a handle on them. Get it? They are not pumped. They are sucked in.

SIMV is most commonly used as the first step to "wean" patients off the ventilator. It gets them started breathing on their own. But they have to breathe on their own for the extra breaths. They have to work to get the extra air.

PEEP/CPAP

For learning purposes PEEP and CPAP are the **same**.

To explain PEEP and CPAP we're going to visualize our lungs as one alveolus that looks like a balloon. On inspiration it fills up with air and the higher pressure inside causes the gas inside to diffuse to the blood.

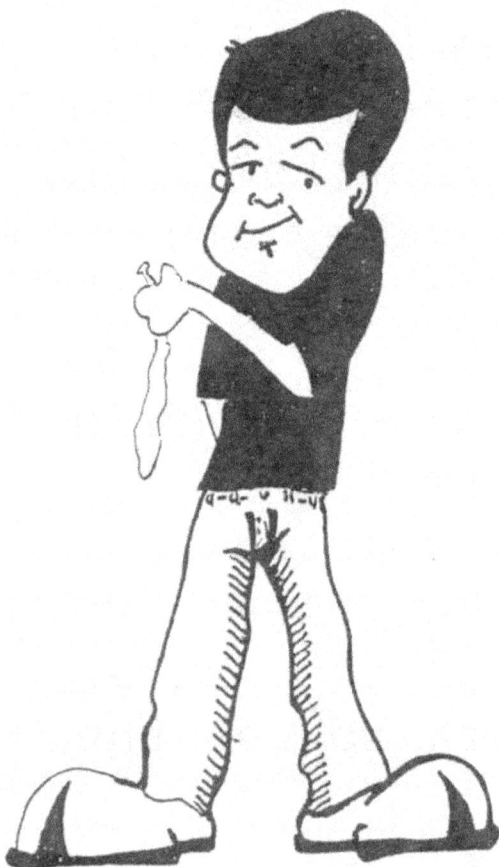

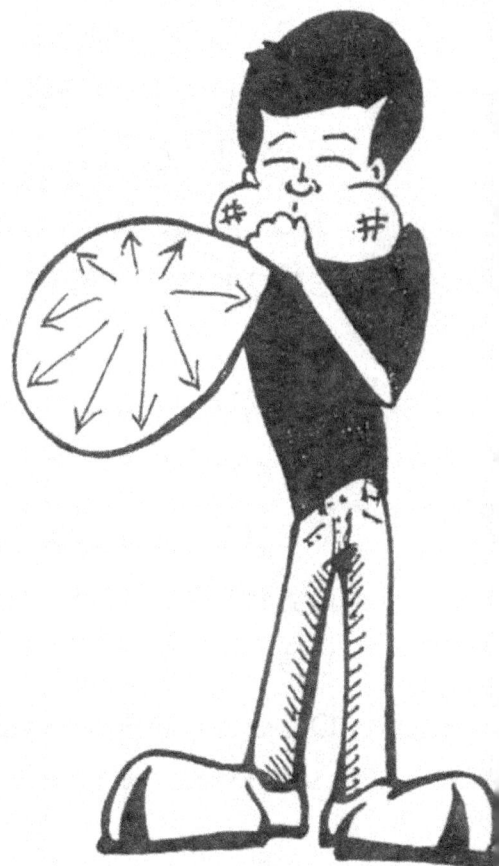

PEEP (Positive End Expiratory Pressure) is a constant small pressure that keeps the alveoli slightly inflated. There are generally two reasons for PEEP/CPAP. Number one is that the small constant pressure improves oxygenation and number two is that it prevents the possibility of collapse.

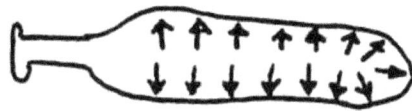

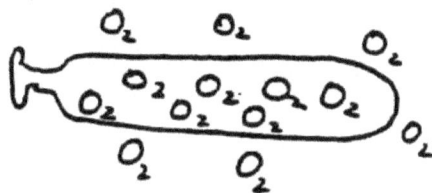

#1

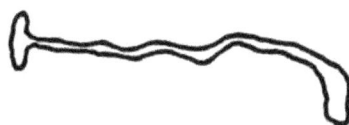

#2

Positive end expiratory pressure prevents the alveoli from collapsing at the end of the breathing cycle. By keeping the alveoli inflated oxygen pressure is maintained and oxygenation of the blood improved.

Let's look at an alveolus as the patient exhales and we'll look at the pressure gauge on the ventilator.

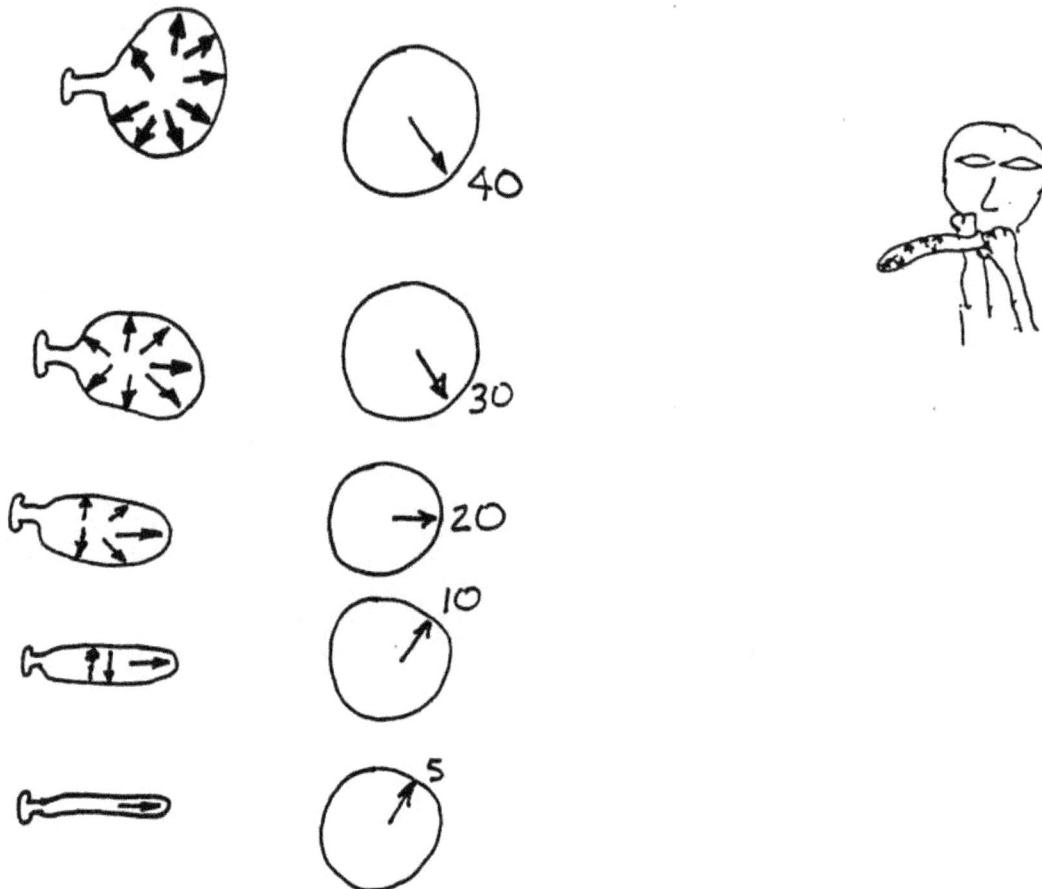

At the end of expiration the alveolus still has positive pressure. Hence the name positive end expiratory pressure. You can tell by looking at the pressure gauge what the PEEP is. The machine settings will also tell you. The pressure does not go below what the PEEP is set at.

Pressure Support

To understand pressure support, try breathing through a straw. It takes a lot of work.

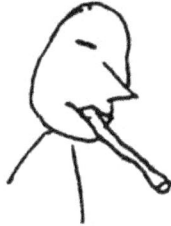

Pressure support adds pressure to the air the patient is inhaling. It lasts as long as the patient is inhaling.

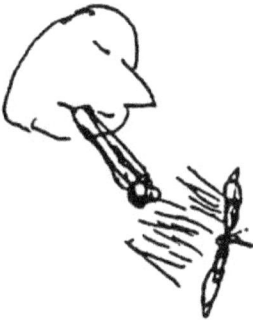

Pressure support does not deliver a set volume, like this pump does.

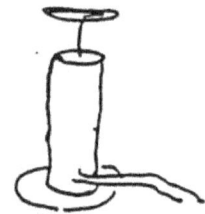

It just gives a boost while the patient is inhaling - like a fan would.

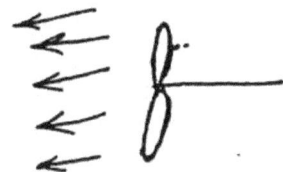

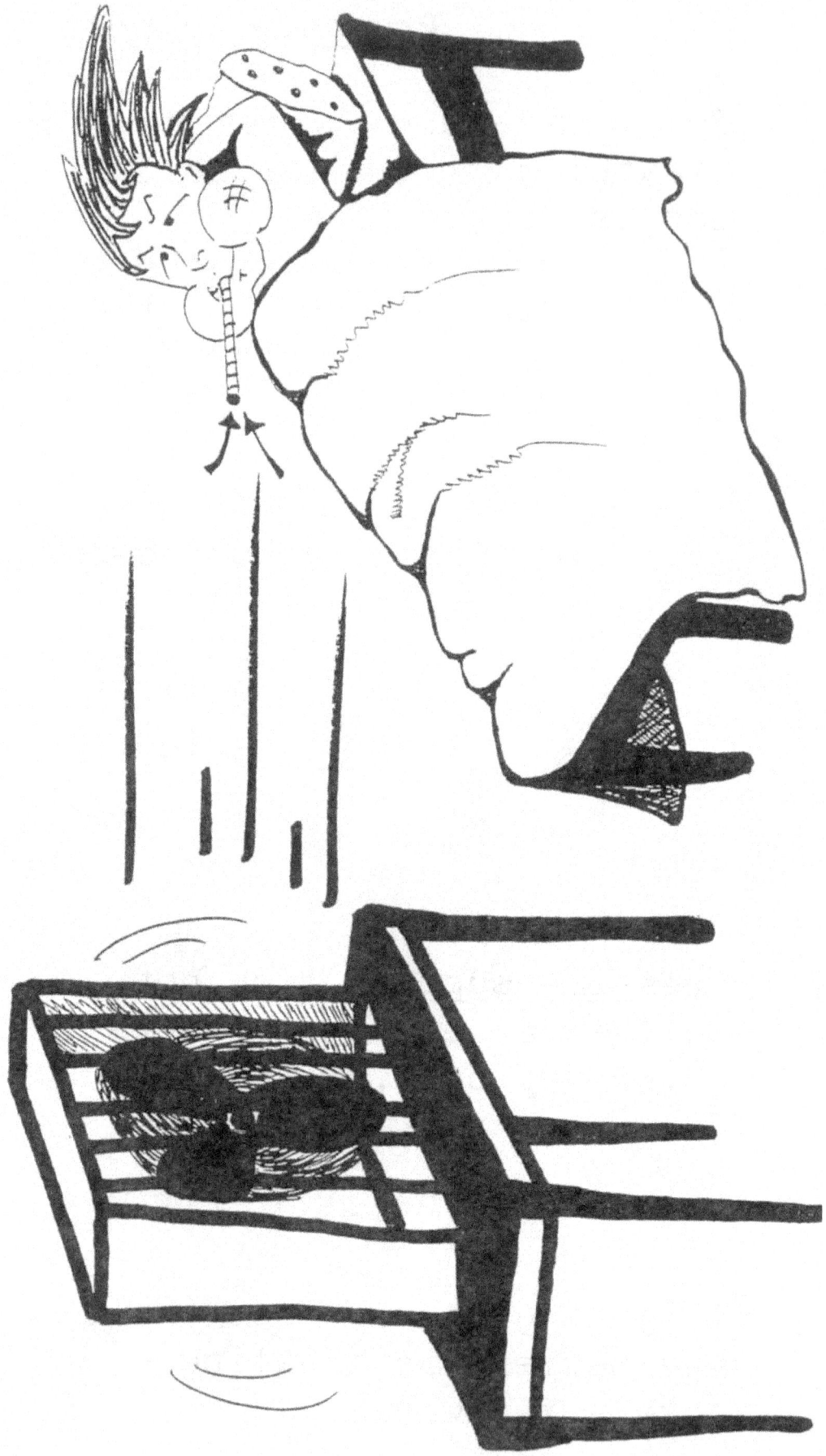

PRESSURE SUPPORT

Example #1

Here is a great example of arterial blood gases and ventilators.

The patient had been brought into the emergency room with respiratory and cardiac arrest. He was intubated the first night. Vent settings were:

FiO_2 50%   AC 20   TV 750   PEEP 5

The next morning ABG's were:

pH 7.64 pCO_2 22 pO_2 238

That means two things. First, he is breathing too often. You can tell that by the alkalotic pH and low pCO_2. Second, he is getting too much oxygen.

You could reduce the oxygen two ways; by lowering the rate and reducing the oxygen content FiO_2. By lowering the rate the patient would blow off less CO_2, which would raise pCO_2 and lower pH.

The pulmonologist changed the vent settings to:

SIMV 12   FiO$_2$ 35   PS 15
The ABG's drawn an hour later after the changes were:

pH 7.48   pCO$_2$ 35   pO$_2$ 112   bicarb 26

The ventilator showed that the patient's respiratory rate was 12, so he still wasn't breathing on his own. By reducing the respiratory rate to 12 it brought the pCO$_2$ up to 35 and the pH down to almost normal. By reducing the rate it also brought down the pO$_2$. But lowering the FiO$_2$ was a much bigger driver of the lower oxygen pressure.

Example #2

Here is a problem that shows a feature of assist control.

The patient was in the unit. She had been found unresponsive and had a long history of emphysema. On a not surprisingly ventilator, the settings were:

SIMV 12   TV 700   PS 12

However, her respiration's were 32, her heart rate was 120 and her O_2 saturation was 97.

The doctor felt she was expending too much energy to breathe. So he changed the SIMV to assist control 10. That way almost all of the energy to breathe would be provided by the machine. Shortly after the changes were made her respirations decreased to 13 and her heart rate decreased to 102. From the resp rate of 13 you see she was only initiating 3 breaths and the machine was providing the full tidal volume. Expending less energy dropped her heart rate to 102.

Example #3

Here is a good ventilator and lung example. The patient had an end stage COPD.

You see vent settings at:

TV 750   AC 20   FiO2 80%   PEEP +15

The gases come back at:

pH 7.31   pCO2 55   pO2 55   HCO3 27

Obviously, the first thing is to improve the O_2 so they change the FiO2 to 100%. Then the gases come back:

pH 7.30   CO2 60   PO2 93   HCO3 29

The major change is a higher pO2. 100% FiO2 in a normal person would produce a PO2 of 500. The PEEP of +15 was the other mechanism for delivering oxygen. Anything higher would likely cause barotrauma.

You will also notice that the respiratory acidosis did not change. The only way to do that would be to increase the respiratory rate and blow off more CO_2.

Alarms

Obviously alarms are quite important in the study of ventilators. Here are the most common alarm situations.

High Inspiratory Pressure

The "high inspiratory pressure" alarm means the ventilator is trying to deliver the set volume and is encountering resistance.

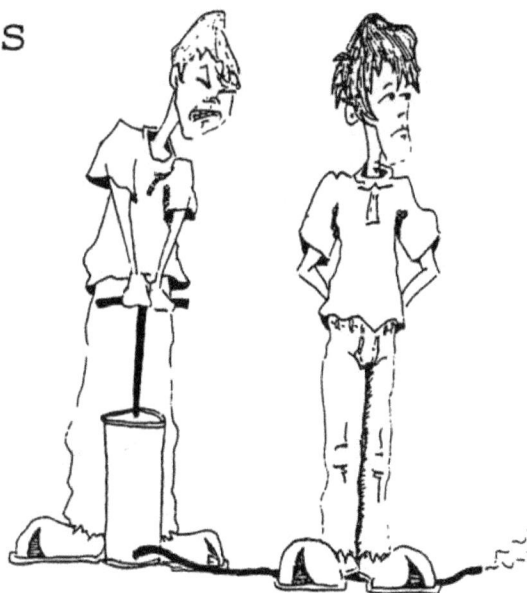

It could be the patient biting on the E.T. (endotracheal) tube. A bite block or sedation could solve that. Worst case would be a mucus plug that has obstructed the flow. For that you would suction the patient, probably with lavage. And if that didn't work you would likely consider an Ambu bag.

Low Inspiratory Pressure

Low Inspiratory Pressure is the machine saying, "It can't be this easy, there's gotta be a catch." That usually means it's become disconnected – which is very bad.

High Inspiratory Rate

High Inspiratory Rate is pretty obvious. It means the patient is breathing quite rapidly. Pain or agitation might be a reason. If the patient was breathing rapidly on IMV it might mean they need to be changed to assist control. That way they would expend less energy.

Low Mechanical Volume

Low Mechanical Volume means the ventilator could not deliver the set volume. If the patient were to cough and trigger the high pressure limit, that could result in a momentary low mechanical volume because the machine did not deliver the full breath. A worse situation would be a leak that was not big enough, set off the "low inspiratory pressure" alarm but it was big enough to drain off significant amounts of air.

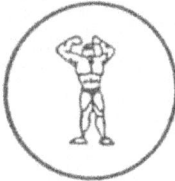
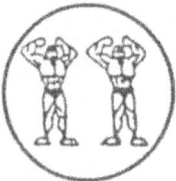
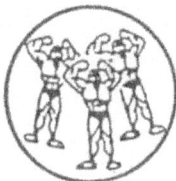
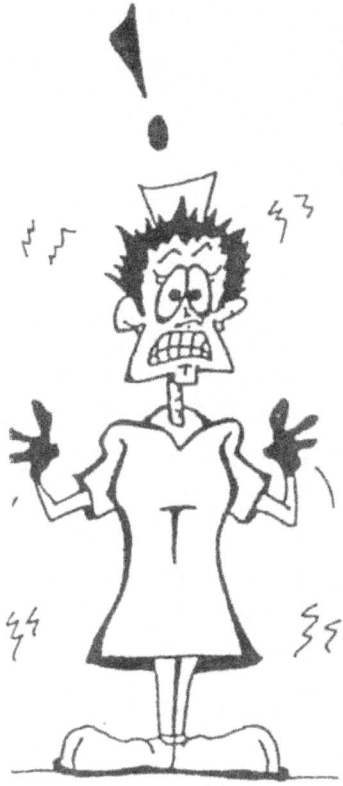
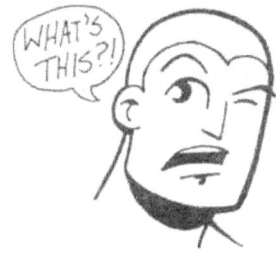

MEDICAL JOKES

Cardiac Joke: What do you get when you spill a urinal?
Answer: see bottom of page

Immunology Joke: "I'm allergic to lasix. It makes me pee."

Hematology Joke: A vampire goes into a blood bank and asks for one unit of packed red cells and one unit of fresh frozen plasma. The phlebotomist yells back to the tech, "Gimme a Blud and a Blud Lite."

Otolaryngology Joke. For otitis media the doctor ordered "corticosporin drops in the R ear QID" The pharmacist called back to say corticosporin doesn't come in suppository form.

Orthopedic Joke (told by an infectious disease doctor): What do you need to do to pass the orthopedic boards? Be able to bench 200 pounds and spell Ancef.

Urology Joke: The doctor is doing a prostate exam. The guy yells, "That hurts!"
The doctor says," I'm using two fingers."
"Why?"
"I want a second opinion."

Infectious Disease Joke: How do you get a Kleenex to dance? Put a little boogie in it.

C.V. Joke: Did you hear about the two red blood cells who loved in vein?

To impress someone try saying, a gram of acetaminocin instead of two extra strength Tylenols.

G.I. Cartoon: There is a doctor, a nurse and a patient. The patient is draped and in the jack knife position presumabley for a sigmoidoscopy.. The nurse is holding a tray with a bottle of beer. The doctor with an angry look says, "No, I said I wanted a butt light."

I.C.U. Cartoon: There is a patient in an I.C.U. bed with monitors , dynamaps, oxygen, and all the familiar paraphanalia. He is talking on the phone saying, "Bells are ringing and the T.V.has a straight line."

A guy goes in to see a doctor. He touches his head and says, every time I touch it here it hurts." He touches his stomach and says the same thing. He touches his knee and repeats it again. The doctor examines him and says, "Your finger is broken."

Answer to cardiology joke: You get a Pee Wave

Plastic Surgery: During routine surgery a woman goes into cardiac arrest. After superhuman efforts and being apparently dead she miraculously recovers. During this ordeal she has an out-of-body experience in which she talks to God. God tells her she get forty more years to live and she should make the most of it be striving to be her best. From that she concludes she should improve her appearance and has liposuction, breast augmentation and a face lift. As she is leaving the hospital a bus hits her and instantly kills her. When she gets to heaven she asks God," What's this all about? You said…" God interrupts, "I didn't recognize you."

Surgery: How does a surgeon change a light bulb? They Just hold it in the socket and stand still. The earth revolves around them.

Psychiatry: How many psychiatrists does it take to change a light bulb?
Only one. But first, the light bulb has to want to change.

A man on a crowded bus a man sees a woman with grocery bags and two small children. He gets up to give her his seat and helps her with the bags.
"Thank you. You're sweet" she says.
"I know. I'm diabetic."
Thanks to Dr. Murray Miller, an endocrinologist, for that one.

How do you tell the difference between an oral thermometer and a rectal thermometer? The taste.

Do you have any good, clean medical jokes? If you do, please send it to me. If I include it on this list, I will give you a copy of any one of my books. Also please specify whether you want your name included as the contributor – or would like to remain anonymous. Please send jokes to Malcolm Rosenberg, P.O. Box 770793, Coral Springs FL 33077 and tell me which book you want. Simplified Arterial Blood Gases, Simplified Ventilators, Simplified Hemodynamics, Drug Calculations for Nurses Who Hate Numbers, or Making the Patients Laugh.

Simplified Ventilators ©1996

Retail: $7.95

ISBN 0-9725483-2-7

9780972548328

0 700814 498009

7 00814 49800 9

www.ingramcontent.com/pod-product-compliance
Lightning Source LLC
Chambersburg PA
CBHW051431200326
41520CB00023B/7438